The Fastest Keto Air Fryer Recipe Book

Super Fast and Delicious Recipes to Boost your Health

Rudy Kent

© **Copyright 2020 - All rights reserved.**

The content contained within this book may not be reproduced, duplicated or transmitted without direct written permission from the author or the publisher.

Under no circumstances will any blame or legal responsibility be held against the publisher, or author, for any damages, reparation, or monetary loss due to the information contained within this book. Either directly or indirectly.

Legal Notice:

This book is copyright protected. This book is only for personal use. You cannot amend, distribute, sell, use, quote or paraphrase any part, or the content within this book, without the consent of the author or publisher.

Disclaimer Notice:

Please note the information contained within this document is for educational and entertainment purposes only. All effort has been executed to present accurate, up to date, and reliable, complete information. No warranties of any kind are declared or implied. Readers acknowledge that the author is not engaging in the rendering of legal, financial, medical or professional advice. The content within this book has been derived from various sources. Please consult a licensed professional before attempting any techniques outlined in this book.

By reading this document, the reader agrees that under no circumstances is the author responsible for any losses, direct or indirect, which are incurred as a result of the use of information contained within this document, including, but not limited to, — errors, omissions, or inaccuracies.

Introduction

What's the difference between an air fryer and deep fryer? Air fryers bake food at a high temperature with a high-powered fan, while deep fryers cook food in a vat of oil that has been heated up to a specific temperature. Both cook food quickly, but an air fryer requires practically zero preheat time while a deep fryer can take upwards of 10 minutes. Air fryers also require little to no oil and deep fryers require a lot that absorb into the food. Food comes out crispy and juicy in both appliances, but don't taste the same, usually because deep fried foods are coated in batter that cook differently in an air fryer vs a deep fryer. Battered foods needs to be sprayed with oil before cooking in an air fryer to help them color and get crispy, while the hot oil soaks into the batter in a deep fryer. Flour-based batters and wet batters don't cook well in an air fryer, but they come out very well in a deep fryer.

The ketogenic diet is one such example. The diet calls for a very small number of carbs to be eaten. This means food such as rice, pasta, and other starchy vegetables like potatoes are off the menu. Even relaxed versions of the keto diet minimize carbs to a large extent and this compromises the goals of many dieters. They end up having to exert large amounts of willpower to follow the diet. This doesn't do them any favors since willpower is like a muscle. At some point, it tires and this is when the dieter goes right back to their old pattern of eating. I have personal experience with this. In terms of health benefits, the keto diet offers the most. The reduction of carbs forces your body to mobilize fat and this results in automatic fat loss and better health.

Feel free to mix and match the recipes you see in here and play around with them. Eating is supposed to be fun! Unfortunately, we've associated fun eating with unhealthy food. This doesn't have to be the case. The air fryer, combined with the Mediterranean diet, will make your mealtimes fun-filled again and full of taste. There's no grease and messy cleanups to deal with anymore. Are you excited yet?

You should be! You're about to embark on a journey full of air fried goodness!

Table of Contents

Introduction 5
- Chicken Stuffed Poblanos 15
- Thai Meatballs 17
- Cheese Herb Zucchini 19
- Delicious Spinach Dip 21
- Cauliflower Hummus 23
- Spicy Mixed Nuts 25
- Tasty Cauliflower Bites 27
- Crab Dip 29
- Broccoli Cheese Balls 31
- Simple Parmesan Zucchini Bites 35
- Yummy Chicken Dip 37
- Roasted Cauliflower Florets 39
- Healthy Carrots Chips 41
- Herb Olives 43
- Healthy Mixed Nuts 45
- Chicken Cheese Dip 47
- Crispy Cauliflower Florets 49
- Goat Cheese Dip 51
- Mexican Cheese Dip 53
- Air Fry Pecans 55
- Roasted Nuts 59
- Cheese Pesto Jalapeno Poppers 61
- Italian-Style Tomato Chips 63

Italian-Style Tomato-Parmesan Crisps 65
Root Vegetable Chips with Dill Mayonnaise 69
Greek-Style Zucchini Rounds 71
Crunchy Wontons with Sausage and Peppers 73
Sweet Potato Chips with Chili Mayo 75
Prosciutto Stuffed Jalapeños 77
Hot Roasted Cauliflower Florets 79
Apple Chips with Walnuts 81
Easy Mexican Elote 83
Classic Jiaozi Chinese Dumplings 85
Mexican-Style Corn on the Cob with Bacon 87
Mini Plantain Cups 89
Sweet Potato Fries with Spicy Dip 91
The Best Calamari Appetizer 93
The Best Party Mix Ever 95
Cocktail Sausage and Veggies on a Stick 97
Red Beet Chips with Pizza Sauce 99
Fried Pickle Chips with Greek Yogurt Dip 101
Parmesan Squash Chips 103
Hot Paprika Bacon Deviled Eggs 105
Kid-Friendly Mozzarella Sticks 107

Healthy Onion Rings

Preparation Time:

10 minutes

Cooking Time:

10 minutes

Serve: 3

Ingredients:

1eggs, lightly beaten
2 large onions, peel & cut into
1-inch slices
1/2 tsp garlic powder
1 tsp paprika
2 tsp Italian seasoning
1 1/2 cups almond flour
1/2 tsp sea salt

Directions:

1.In a small bowl, add eggs and whisk well. In a shallow bowl, mix together almond flour, Italian seasoning, paprika, garlic powder, and sea salt.

2.Dip onion slice into the egg then coat with almond flour mixture.

3.Place breaded onion slices onto the parchment-lined plate and place it in the refrigerator for 30 minutes.

4.Place the cooking tray in the air fryer basket. Place piece of parchment paper into the air fryer basket. Select Air Fry mode. Set time to 10 minutes and temperature 380 F then press START.

5.The air fryer display will prompt you to ADD FOOD once the temperature is reached then place onion slices onto the parchment paper in the air fryer basket.

6.Spray onion slices with cooking spray. Turn onion slices halfway through. Serve and enjoy.

Crispy Parmesan Asparagus Fries

Preparation Time:

10 minutes

Cooking Time:

12 minutes

Serve:

4

Ingredients:

1 eggs, lightly beaten
16 asparagus, trim
2-inches of bottom
1/2 cup parmesan cheese, grated
1 tbsp garlic powder
1/2 tbsp paprika
2 cups pork rinds, crushed
1 tbsp olive oil
2 tbsp heavy cream
1 tsp pepper

Directions:

1. In a shallow dish, whisk eggs with olive oil, and heavy cream.

2. On a plate, mix together crushed pork rinds, pepper, paprika, garlic powder, and parmesan cheese. Dip asparagus in egg then coat with pork rind mixture.

3. Place the cooking tray in the air fryer basket. Place piece of parchment paper into the air fryer basket.

4.Select Bake mode. Set time to 12 minutes and temperature 400 F then press START.

5.The air fryer display will prompt you to ADD FOOD once the temperature is reached then place coated asparagus onto the parchment paper in the air fryer basket. Serve and enjoy

Crab Stuffed Jalapenos

Preparation Time:

10 minutes

Cooking Time:

20 minutes

Serve: 10

Ingredients:

8 oz lump crab meat
10 jalapenos, cut in half & remove seeds
2 green onions, sliced
3 bacon slices, cooked and crumbled
3/4 cup cheddar cheese, shredded
1/4 tsp garlic powder
1/2 tsp Cajun seasoning
4 oz cream cheese, softened

Directions:

1. In a bowl, mix together crab meat, green onions, bacon, cheese, garlic powder, cajun seasoning, and cream cheese.

2. Stuff crab meat mixture into each jalapeno half. Place the cooking tray in the air fryer basket. Select Bake mode.

3. Set time to 20 minutes and temperature 375 F then press START.

4. The air fryer display will prompt you to ADD FOOD once the temperature is reached then place stuff jalapenos in the air fryer basket. Serve and enjoy.

Chicken Stuffed Poblanos

Preparation Time:

10 minutes

Cooking Time:

15 minutes

Serve: 6

Ingredients:

3 poblano pepper, cut in half & remove seeds
2 oz cheddar cheese, grated
1 1/2 cups spinach artichoke dip
1 cup chicken breast, cooked & chopped

Directions:

1. In a bowl, mix together chicken, spinach artichoke dip, and half cheddar cheese.

2. Stuff chicken mixture into each poblano pepper half.

3. Place the cooking tray in the air fryer basket. Line air fryer basket with parchment paper.

4. Select Air Fry mode. Set time to 15 minutes and temperature 350 F then press START.

5. The air fryer display will prompt you to ADD FOOD once the temperature is reached then place stuff poblano pepper onto the parchment paper in the air fryer basket.

6.Sprinkle remaining cheese on top of stuff peppers. Serve and enjoy.

Thai Meatballs

Preparation Time:

10 minutes

Cooking Time:

20 minutes

Serve: 6

Ingredients:

2 eggs, lightly beaten
2 lbs ground turkey
1 tsp crushed red pepper
2 tbsp lemongrass, chopped
3 tbsp fish sauce
3 garlic cloves, minced
1/2 cup fresh basil, chopped
3/4 cup scallions, chopped
1 cup almond flour

Directions:

1. Add ground turkey in the mixing bowl. Add remaining ingredients and mix until well combined.

2. Make small balls from the turkey mixture. Place the cooking tray in the air fryer basket. Line air fryer basket with parchment paper.

3. Select Bake mode. Set time to 20 minutes and temperature 400 F then press START.

4.The air fryer display will prompt you to ADD FOOD once the temperature is reached then place meatballs onto the parchment paper in the air fryer basket. Turn meatballs halfway through. Serve and enjoy.

Cheese Herb Zucchini

Preparation Time:

10 minutes

Cooking Time:

15 minutes

Serve: 4

Ingredients:

4 zucchini, quartered lengthwise
2 tbsp fresh parsley, chopped
1/2 tsp dried oregano
1/2 tsp dried thyme
1/2 cup parmesan cheese, grated
2 tbsp olive oil
1/4 tsp garlic powder
1/2 tsp dried basil
Pepper Salt

Directions:

1. In a small bowl, mix together parmesan cheese, garlic powder, basil, oregano, thyme, pepper, and salt. Place the cooking tray in the air fryer basket.

2. Line air fryer basket with parchment paper. Select Bake mode. Set time to 15 minutes and temperature 350 F then press START.

3. The air fryer display will prompt you to ADD FOOD once the temperature is reached then arrange zucchini onto the parchment paper in the air fryer basket.

4. Drizzle with oil and sprinkle with parmesan cheese mixture. Garnish with parsley and serve.

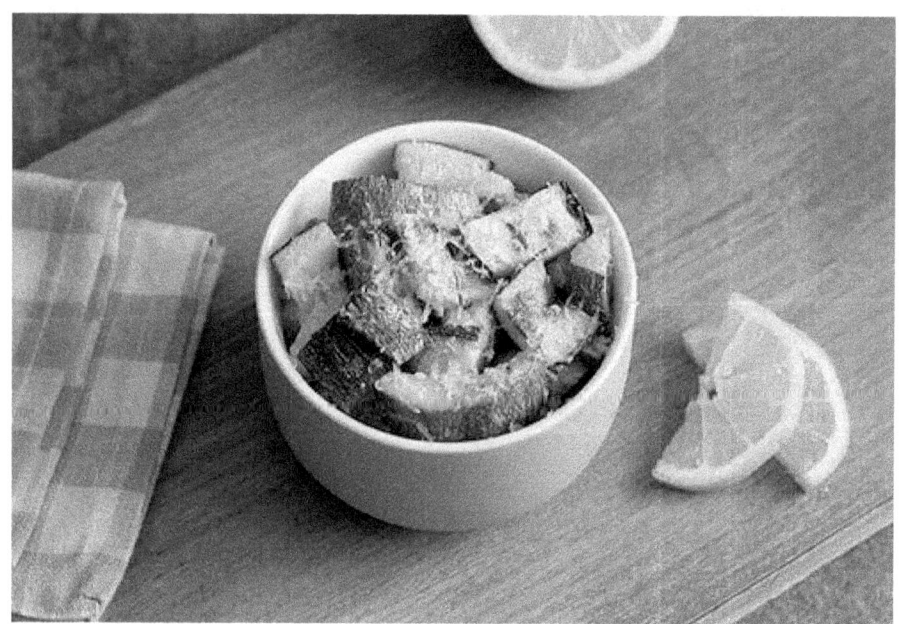

Delicious Spinach Dip

Preparation Time:

10 minutes

Cooking Time:

20 minutes

Serve: 12

Ingredients:

3 oz frozen spinach, defrosted & chopped
1 cup cheddar cheese, shredded
8 oz cream cheese
1 cup Asiago cheese, shredded
1 cup sour cream
1 tsp salt

Directions:

1. Add all ingredients into the mixing bowl and mix until well combined. Transfer mixture into the baking dish.

2. Cover dish with foil. Select Bake mode. Set time to 20 minutes and temperature 350 F then press START.

3. The air fryer display will prompt you to ADD FOOD once the temperature is reached then baking dish in the air fryer basket. Serve and enjoy

Cauliflower Hummus

Preparation Time:

10 minutes

Cooking Time:

35 minutes

Serve: 8

Ingredients:

1 cauliflower head, cut into florets
3 tbsp olive oil
1/2 tsp ground cumin
1 tsp garlic, chopped
2 tbsp fresh lemon juice
1/3 cup tahini
Pepper Salt

Directions:

1. Place the cooking tray in the air fryer basket. Line air fryer basket with parchment paper. Select Bake mode.

2. Set time to 35 minutes and temperature 400 F then press START. The air fryer display will prompt you to ADD FOOD once the temperature is reached then spread cauliflower onto the parchment paper in the air fryer basket.

3. Transfer roasted cauliflower into the food processor along with remaining ingredients and process until smooth. Serve and enjoy

Spicy Mixed Nuts

Preparation Time:

10 minutes

Cooking Time:

4 minutes

Serve: 2

Ingredients:

1cup mixed nuts
1 tsp chili powder
1 tsp ground cumin
1 tbsp olive oil
1 tsp pepper
1 tsp salt

Directions:

1. In a bowl, add all ingredients and toss well. Place the cooking tray in the air fryer basket. Line air fryer basket with parchment paper.

2. Select Air Fry mode. Set time to 4 minutes and temperature 350 F then press START.

3. The air fryer display will prompt you to ADD FOOD once the temperature is reached then place mixed nuts onto the parchment paper in the air fryer basket. Serve and enjoy.

Tasty Cauliflower Bites

Preparation Time:

10 minutes

Cooking Time:

15 minutes

Serve: 4

Ingredients:

1 lb cauliflower florets
1/2 tsp dried rosemary
1 1/2 tsp garlic powder
1 tbsp olive oil
1 tsp sesame seeds
1 tsp ground coriander
Pepper Salt

Directions:

1. Place the cooking tray in the air fryer basket. Line air fryer basket with parchment paper. Select Bake mode.

2. Set time to 15 minutes and temperature 400 F then press START.

3. The air fryer display will prompt you to ADD FOOD once the temperature is reached then spread cauliflower florets onto the parchment paper in the air fryer basket. Serve and enjoy.

Crab Dip

Preparation Time:

10 minutes

Cooking Time:

7 minutes

Serve: 4

Ingredients:

1 cup crab, cooked
2 tbsp fresh parsley, chopped
2 tbsp fresh lemon juice
2 tbsp hot sauce
2 cups Jalapeno jack cheese, grated
1/2 cup green onions, sliced
1/4 cup mayonnaise
1 tsp pepper
1/2 tsp salt

Directions:

1. Add all ingredients except parsley and lemon juice in the 6-inch baking dish and mix well. Select Air Fry mode.

2. Set time to 7 minutes and temperature 400 F then press START.

3. The air fryer display will prompt you to ADD FOOD once the temperature is reached then place the baking dish in the air fryer basket.

4. Remove dish from air fryer. Add parsley and lemon juice. Mix well. Serve and enjoy.

Broccoli Cheese Balls

Preparation Time:

10 minutes

Cooking Time:

30 minutes

Serve: 20

Ingredients:

1 eggs
1/4 cup onion, minced
1/2 cup almond flour
2 cups broccoli florets
1 tsp Italian seasoning
1 garlic clove, minced
1 cup cheddar cheese, shredded
Pepper Salt

Directions:

1. Steam broccoli florets in boiling water until tender. Drain well and chopped.

2. In a large bowl, mix together broccoli, eggs, cheese, almond flour, onion, garlic, and spices until well combined.

3. Make small balls from the mixture. Place the cooking tray in the air fryer basket. Line air fryer basket with parchment paper.

4. Select Bake mode. Set time to 30 minutes and temperature 400 F then press START.

5.The air fryer display will prompt you to ADD FOOD once the temperature is reached then place broccoli balls onto the parchment paper in the air fryer basket. Serve and enjoy.

Pepperoni Chips

Preparation Time:

10 minutes

Cooking Time:

10 minutes

Serve: 2

Ingredients:

1 oz pepperoni
4 tbsp mozzarella cheese, shredded
2 tbsp parmesan cheese, grated
1/2 tsp Italian seasoning

Directions:

1. Place the cooking tray in the air fryer basket. Line air fryer basket with parchment paper.

2. Select Bake mode. Set time to 10 minutes and temperature 400 F then press START.

3. The air fryer display will prompt you to ADD FOOD once the temperature is reached then arrange pepperoni onto the parchment paper in the air fryer basket.

4. Sprinkle parmesan cheese, Italian seasoning, and mozzarella cheese over pepperoni. Serve and enjoy.

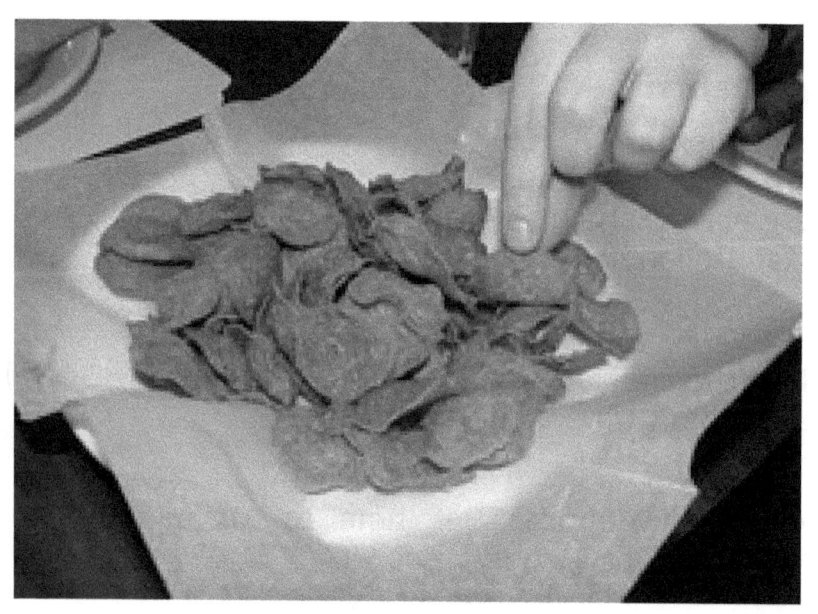

Simple Parmesan Zucchini Bites

Preparation Time:

10 minutes

Cooking Time:

15 minutes

Serve: 4

Ingredients:

1egg
1/2 cup parmesan cheese, grated
2 cups zucchini, grated
1/4 cup cilantro, chopped
Pepper Salt

Directions:

1. In a bowl, mix together zucchini, cilantro, cheese, egg, pepper, and salt. Pour mixture into the small baking dish.

2. Select Bake mode. Set time to 15 minutes and temperature 400 F then press START.

3. The air fryer display will prompt you to ADD FOOD once the temperature is reached then place the baking dish in the air fryer basket. Serve and enjoy.

Yummy Chicken Dip

Preparation Time:

10 minutes

Cooking Time:

25 minutes

Serve: 6

Ingredients:

1cups chicken, cooked and shredded
1/2 cup sour cream
8 oz cream cheese, softened
4 tbsp hot sauce

Directions:

1. Add all ingredients in a large bowl and mix until well combined.

2. Transfer mixture in a baking dish. Cover dish with foil. Select Bake mode.

3. Set time to 25 minutes and temperature 350 F then press START.

4. The air fryer display will prompt you to ADD FOOD once the temperature is reached then place the baking dish in the air fryer basket. Serve and enjoy.

Roasted Cauliflower Florets

Preparation Time:

10 minutes

Cooking Time:

20 minutes

Serve: 4

Ingredients:

5 cups cauliflower florets
1/2 tsp cumin powder
1/2 tsp garlic powder
1/4 tsp onion powder
1/4 tsp chili powder
1/2 tsp coriander powder
4 tablespoons olive oil
1/2 tsp salt

Directions:

1. Add all ingredients into the large bowl and toss well. Place the cooking tray in the air fryer basket.

2. Line air fryer basket with parchment paper. Select Air Fry mode.

3. Set time to 20 minutes and temperature 400 F then press START.

4. The air fryer display will prompt you to ADD FOOD once the temperature is reached then place cauliflower florets onto the parchment paper in the air fryer basket.

Serve and enjoy.

Healthy Carrots Chips

Preparation Time:

10 minutes

Cooking Time:

12 minutes

Serve: 4

Ingredients:

12 oz carrot chips
1 tbsp olive oil
1/4 tsp paprika
1/4 tsp pepper
1/2 tsp garlic powder
1/2 tsp salt

Directions:

1. Add all ingredients into the bowl and toss well. Place the cooking tray in the air fryer basket.

2. Line air fryer basket with parchment paper. Select Air Fry mode. Set time to 12 minutes and temperature 375 F then press START.

3. The air fryer display will prompt you to ADD FOOD once the temperature is reached then place carrot chips onto the parchment paper in the air fryer basket. Serve and enjoy.

Herb Olives

Preparation Time:

10 minutes

Cooking Time:

5 minutes

Serve: 4

Ingredients:

2 cups olives
1/2 tsp crushed red pepper
2 tsp garlic, minced
2 tbsp olive oil
1/2 tsp dried fennel seeds
1/2 tsp dried oregano
Pepper Salt

Directions:

1.Add olives and remaining ingredients into the mixing bowl and toss to coat well.

2.Place the cooking tray in the air fryer basket. Line air fryer basket with parchment paper.

3.Select Air Fry mode. Set time to 5 minutes and temperature 300 F then press START.

4.The air fryer display will prompt you to ADD FOOD once the temperature is reached then place olives onto the parchment paper in the air fryer basket. Serve and enjoy.

Healthy Mixed Nuts

Preparation Time:

5 minutes

Cooking Time:

20 minutes

Serve: 20

Ingredients:

5 cups mixed nuts
1 tsp paprika
1 tsp onion powder
1 tsp garlic powder
1/4 cup olive oil
1 tsp salt

Directions:

1.Add mixed nuts and remaining ingredients into the mixing bowl and mix well. Place the cooking tray in the air fryer basket.

2.Line air fryer basket with parchment paper. Select Bake mode. Set time to 20 minutes and temperature 325 F then press START.

3.The air fryer display will prompt you to ADD FOOD once the temperature is reached then spread nuts onto the parchment paper in the air fryer basket. Serve and enjoy.

Chicken Cheese Dip

Preparation Time:

10 minutes

Cooking Time:

10 minutes

Serve: 8

Ingredients:

2 cups cheddar cheese, shredded
1 cup ranch dressing
2 can chunk chicken, drained
1 package cream cheese
3/4 cup hot sauce

Directions:

1. Add chicken and hot sauce to the pan and cook for 2 minutes.

2. Add cream and ranch dressing and stir well. Add half cheese and stir until well blended. Transfer chicken mixture to the baking dish and sprinkle the remaining cheese on
top.

3. Cover dish with foil. Select Bake mode. Set time to 10 minutes and temperature 370 F then press START.

4. The air fryer display will prompt you to ADD FOOD once the temperature is reached then place the baking dish in the air fryer basket. Serve and enjoy

Crispy Cauliflower Florets

Preparation Time:

10 minutes

Cooking Time:

15 minutes

Serve: 4

Ingredients:

1 medium cauliflower head, cut into florets
1/2 tsp Italian seasoning
1/4 tsp paprika
1/4 tsp onion powder
1 tbsp garlic, minced
3 tbsp olive oil
Pepper Salt

Directions:

1. In a large bowl, toss cauliflower with remaining ingredients.

2. Place the cooking tray in the air fryer basket. Line air fryer basket with parchment paper. Select Bake mode.

3. Set time to 15 minutes and temperature 400 F then press START.

4. The air fryer display will prompt you to ADD FOOD once the temperature is reached then spread cauliflower florets onto the parchment paper in the air fryer basket. Serve and enjoy.

Goat Cheese Dip

Preparation Time:

10 minutes

Cooking Time:

10 minutes

Serve: 4

Ingredients:

10 oz goat cheese
2 garlic cloves, minced
1/4 tsp sage
1/4 tsp thyme
2 tbsp olive oil
1/4 cup parmesan cheese
Pepper Salt

Directions:

1. Add all ingredients into the food processor and process until just combined. Pour mixture into the prepared baking dish and spread well.

2. Select Bake mode. Set time to 10 minutes and temperature 400 F then press START.

3. The air fryer display will prompt you to ADD FOOD once the temperature is reached then place the baking dish in the air fryer basket. Serve and enjoy.

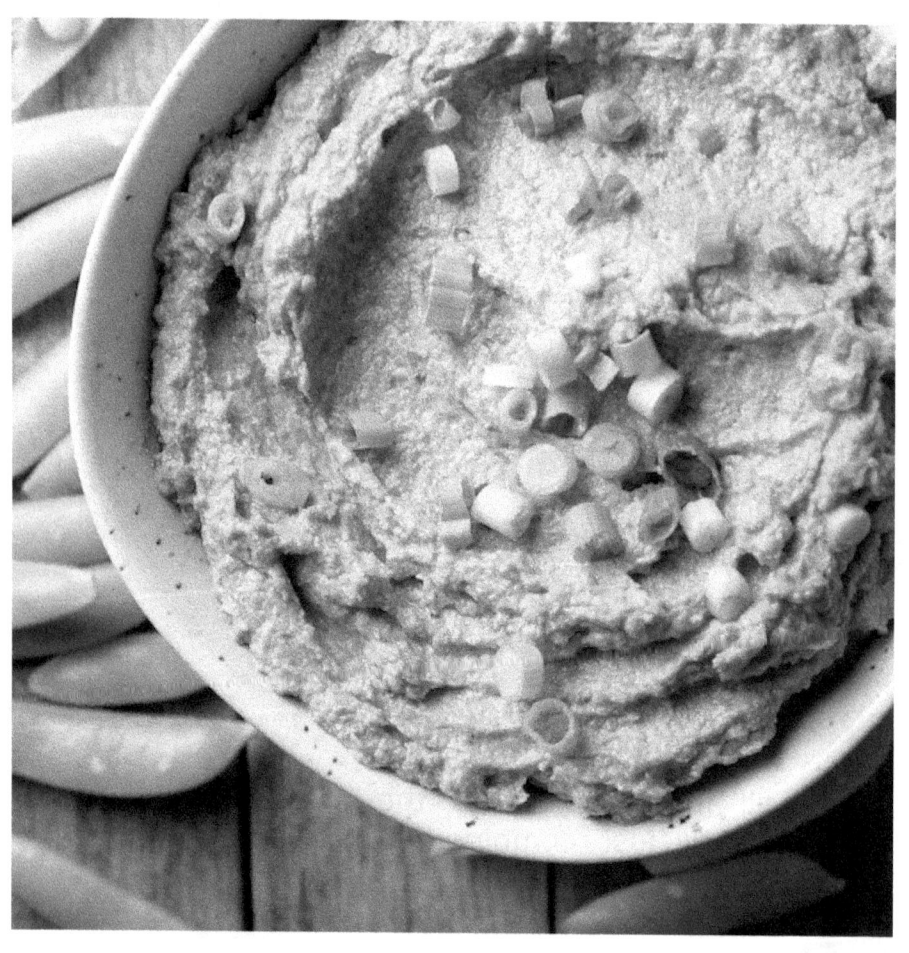

Mexican Cheese Dip

Preparation Time:

10 minutes

Cooking Time:

30 minutes

Serve: 10

Ingredients:

1/2 cup hot salsa
3 cups cheddar cheese, shredded
16 oz cream cheese, softened
1 cup sour cream

Directions:

1. In a bowl, mix together all ingredients until well combined and pour into the baking dish. Cover dish with foil.

2. Select Bake mode. Set time to 30 minutes and temperature 350 F then press START.

3. The air fryer display will prompt you to ADD FOOD once the temperature is reached then place the baking dish in the air fryer basket. Serve and enjoy.

Air Fry Pecans

Preparation Time:

5 minutes

Cooking Time:

6 minutes

Serve: 6

Ingredients:

2 cups pecan halves
1 tbsp butter, melted
1/4 tsp chili powder
Salt

Directions:

1. Add pecans, chili powder, butter, and salt in a mixing bowl and toss well. Place the cooking tray in the air fryer basket.

2. Line air fryer basket with parchment paper. Select Bake mode. Set time to 6 minutes and temperature 400 F then press START.

3. The air fryer display will prompt you to ADD FOOD once the temperature is reached then place pecans onto the parchment paper in the air fryer basket. Serve and enjoy.

Stuffed Mushrooms

Preparation Time:

10 minutes

Cooking Time:

5 minutes

Serve: 3

Ingredients:

12 baby mushrooms
4 bacon slices, cooked and crumbled
4 oz cream cheese
2 tbsp butter, melted
Pepper Salt

Directions:

1. In a small bowl, mix together cream cheese, butter, bacon, pepper, and salt. Stuff cream cheese mixture into the mushrooms.

2. Place the cooking tray in the air fryer basket. Line air fryer basket with parchment paper. Select Bake mode.

3. Set time to 5 minutes and temperature 350 F then press START.

4. The air fryer display will prompt you to ADD FOOD once the temperature is reached then place stuffed mushrooms onto the parchment paper in the air fryer basket. Serve and enjoy.

Roasted Nuts

Preparation Time:

10 minutes

Cooking Time:

15 minutes

Serve: 6

Ingredients:

1 cup cashew nuts
1 cup almonds
1/2 tsp chili powder
1 tbsp olive oil
1/2 tsp salt

Directions

1. In a bowl, toss almonds and cashew with oil, chili powder, and salt. Place the cooking tray in the air fryer basket.

2. Line air fryer basket with parchment paper. Select Bake mode. Set time to 15 minutes and temperature 300 F then press START.

3. The air fryer display will prompt you to ADD FOOD once the temperature is reached then place cashew and almonds onto the parchment paper in the air fryer basket. Serve and enjoy.

Cheese Pesto Jalapeno Poppers

Preparation Time:

10 minutes

Cooking Time:

15 minutes

Serve: 6

Ingredients:

3 jalapeno peppers, halved and remove seeds
3 tbsp basil pesto
1/4 cup cream cheese
1/2 cup mozzarella cheese, shredded

Directions:

1. In a bowl, mix together pesto, shredded cheese, and cream cheese. Stuff pesto cheese mixture into each jalapeno half.

2. Place the cooking tray in the air fryer basket. Line air fryer basket with parchment paper. Select Bake mode. Set time to 15 minutes and temperature 400 F then press START.

3. The air fryer display will prompt you to ADD FOOD once the temperature is reached then place stuffed jalapeno halves onto the parchment paper in the air fryer basket. Serve and enjoy.

Italian-Style Tomato Chips

Cooking Time:

20 minutes

Serve: 2

Ingredients:

2 tomatoes, cut into thick rounds
1 teaspoon extra-virgin olive oil
Sea salt and fresh ground pepper, to taste
1 teaspoon Italian seasoning mix
¼ cup Romano cheese, grated

Directions:

1. Preheat air fryer to 350 F. Toss the tomato sounds with remaining ingredients. Transfer the tomato rounds to the cooking basket without overlapping.

2. Cook your tomato rounds in the preheated Air Fryer for 5 minutes. Flip them over and cook an additional 5 minutes. Work with batches. Serve warm.

Italian-Style Tomato-Parmesan Crisps

Cooking Time:

20 minutes

Serve: 4

Ingredients:

4 Roma tomatoes, sliced
2 tablespoons olive oil
Sea salt and white pepper, to taste
1 teaspoon Italian seasoning mix
4 tablespoons Parmesan cheese, grated

Directions:

1. Preheat air fryer to 350 F. Generously grease the Air Fryer basket with nonstick cooking oil.

2. Toss the sliced tomatoes with the remaining ingredients. Transfer them to the cooking basket without overlapping.

3. Cook in the preheated Air Fryer for 5 minutes. Shake the cooking basket and cook an additional 5 minutes. Work in batches.

4. Serve with Mediterranean aioli for dipping, if desired. Enjoy!

Bruschetta with Fresh Tomato and Basil

Cooking Time:

15 minutes

Serve: 3

Ingredients:

½ Italian bread, sliced
2 garlic cloves, peeled
2 tablespoons extra-virgin olive oil
2 ripe tomatoes, chopped
1 teaspoon dried oregano
Salt, to taste
8 fresh basil leaves, roughly chopped

Directions:

1.Place the bread slices on the lightly greased Air Fryer grill pan. Bake at 370 degrees F for 3 minutes. Cut a clove of garlic in half and rub over one side of the toast; brush with olive oil.

2.Add the chopped tomatoes. Sprinkle with oregano and salt. Increase the temperature to 380 degrees F. Cook in the preheated Air Fryer for 3 minutes more. Garnish with fresh basil and serve. Serve and enjoy!

Root Vegetable Chips with Dill Mayonnaise

Cooking Time:

40 minutes

Serve: 4

Ingredients:

½ pound red beetroot, julienned
½ pound golden beetroot, julienned
¼ pound carrot, julienned
Sea salt and ground black pepper, to taste
1 teaspoon olive oil
½ cup mayonnaise
1 teaspoon garlic, minced
¼ teaspoon dried dill weed

Directions:

1. Toss your veggies with salt, black pepper and olive oil. Arrange the veggie chips in a single layer in the Air Fryer cooking basket.

2. Cook the veggie chips in the preheated Air Fryer at 340 degrees F for 20 minutes; tossing the basket occasionally to ensure even cooking. Work with two batches.

3. Meanwhile, mix the mayonnaise, garlic and dill until well combined. Serve the vegetable chips with the mayo sauce on the side. and serve.

Greek-Style Zucchini Rounds

Cooking Time:

15 minutes

Serve: 3

Ingredients:

½ pound zucchini, cut into thin rounds
1 teaspoon extra-virgin olive oil
½ teaspoon dried sage, crushed
½ teaspoon oregano
¼ teaspoon ground bay leaf Coarse
Sea salt and ground black pepper, to taste

Greek dipping sauce:

½ cup Greek yogurt
½ teaspoon fresh lemon juice
2 tablespoons mayonnaise
½ teaspoon garlic, pressed

Directions:

1. Toss the zucchini rounds with olive oil and spices and place them in the Air Fryer cooking basket.

2. Cook in the preheated Air Fryer at 400 degrees F for 10 minutes; shaking the basket halfway through the cooking time.

3. Let it cool slightly and cook an additional minute or so until crispy and golden brown. Meanwhile, make the sauce by whisking all the sauce ingredients; place the

sauce in the refrigerator until ready to serve. Serve the crispy zucchini rounds with Greek dipping sauce on the side. Serve warm.

Crunchy Wontons with Sausage and Peppers

Cooking Time:

20 minutes

Serve: 3

Ingredients:

20 3-½-inch wonton wrappers
½ pound beef sausage crumbled
1 bell pepper, deveined and chopped
1 teaspoon sesame oil
½ teaspoon granulated garlic
1 tablespoon soy sauce
1 tablespoon rice wine vinegar
1 tablespoon honey
1 teaspoon Sriracha sauce
1 teaspoon sesame seeds, toasted

Directions:

1.Mix the crumbled sausage with the chopped pepper and set it aside. Place wonton wrappers on a clean work surface.

2.Divide the sausage filling between the wrappers. Wet the edge of each wrapper with water, fold the top half over the bottom half and pinch the border to seal.

3.Place the wontons in the cooking basket and brush them with a little bit of olive oil. Cook the wontons at

400 degrees F for 8 minutes.

4.Work with batches. In the meantime, whisk the sauce ingredients and set it aside. Serve the warm wontons with the sauce for dipping. Enjoy!

Sweet Potato Chips with Chili Mayo

Cooking Time:

35 minutes

Serve: 3

Ingredients:

1 sweet potato, cut into 1/8-inch-thick slices
1 teaspoon olive oil
Sea salt and cracked mixed peppercorns, to taste
½ teaspoon turmeric powder
⅓ cup mayonnaise
1 teaspoon granulated garlic
½ teaspoon red chili flakes

Directions:

1. Toss the sweet potato slices with olive oil, salt, cracked peppercorns and turmeric powder.

2. Cook your sweet potatoes at 380 degrees F for 33 to 35 minutes, tossing the basket every 10 minutes to ensure even cooking. Work with batches.

3. Meanwhile, mix the mayonnaise, garlic and red chili flakes to make the sauce. The sweet potato chips will crisp up as it cools. Serve the sweet potato chips with the chili mayo on the side.

Prosciutto Stuffed Jalapeños

Cooking Time:

15 minutes

Serve: 2

Ingredients:

8 fresh jalapeño peppers, deseeded and cut in half lengthwise
4 ounces Ricotta cheese, at room temperature
¼ teaspoon cayenne pepper
½ teaspoon granulated garlic
8 slices prosciutto, chopped

Directions:

1. Place the fresh jalapeño peppers on a clean surface. Mix the remaining ingredients in a bowl; divide the filling between the jalapeño peppers.

2. Transfer the peppers to the Air Fryer cooking basket. Cook the stuffed peppers at 400 degrees F for 15 minutes. Serve and enjoy!

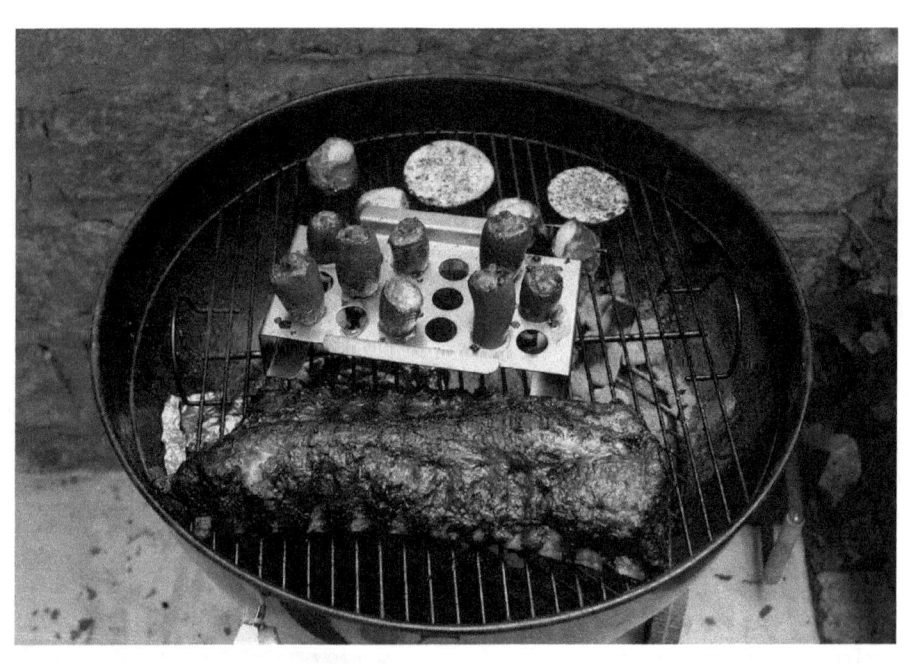

Hot Roasted Cauliflower Florets

Cooking Time:

20 minutes

Serve: 3

Ingredients:

½ cup plain flour
½ teaspoon shallot powder
1 teaspoon garlic powder
¼ teaspoon dried dill weed
½ teaspoon chipotle powder
Sea salt and ground black pepper, to taste
½ cup rice milk
2 tablespoons coconut oil, softened
1 pound cauliflower florets

Directions:

1. In a mixing bowl, thoroughly combine the flour, spices, rice milk and coconut oil. Mix to combine well.

2. Coat the cauliflower florets with the batter and allow the excess batter to drip back into the bowl.

3. Cook the cauliflower florets at 400 degrees F for 12 minutes, shaking the basket once or twice to ensure even browning. Serve with some extra hot sauce, if desired. Enjoy!

Apple Chips with Walnuts

Cooking Time:

35 minutes

Serve: 2

Ingredients:

2 apples, peeled, cored and sliced
½ teaspoon ground cloves
1 teaspoon cinnamon
¼ cup walnuts

Directions:

1. Toss the apple slices with ground cloves and cinnamon.

2. Place the apple slices in the Air Fryer cooking basket and cook at 360 degrees F for 10 minutes or until crisp. Reserve.

3. Then, toast the walnuts at 300 degrees F for 10 minutes; now, shake the basket and cook for another 10 minutes.

4. Chop the walnuts and scatter them over the apple slices and serve.

Easy Mexican Elote

Cooking Time:

10 minutes

Serve: 2

Ingredients:

2 ears of corn, husked
4 tablespoons Mexican crema
4 tablespoons Mexican cheese blend, crumbled
1 teaspoon fresh lime juice
Sea salt and chili powder, to taste
1 tablespoon fresh cilantro, chopped

Directions:

1. Cook the corn in the preheated Air Fryer at 390 degrees F for about 6 minutes. Mix the Mexican crema, Mexican cheese blend, lime juice, salt and chili powder in a bowl.

2. Afterwards, insert a wooden stick into the core as a handle. Rub each ear of corn with the topping mixture. Garnish with fresh chopped cilantro. Serve immediately.

Classic Jiaozi Chinese Dumplings

Cooking Time:

15 minutes

Serve: 2

Ingredients:

½ pound ground pork
1 cup Napa cabbage, shredded
2 scallion stalks, chopped
1 ounce bamboo shoots, shredded
½ teaspoon garlic paste
1 teaspoon fresh ginger, peeled and grated
8 ounces round wheat dumpling

Sauce:

2 tablespoons rice vinegar

¼ cup soy sauce

1 tablespoon ketchup

1 teaspoon deli mustard

1 teaspoon honey

1 teaspoon sesame seeds, lightly toasted

Directions:

1. Cook the pork in a wok that is preheated over medium-high heat; cook until no longer pink and stir in the Napa cabbage, scallions, bamboo shoots, garlic paste and ginger; salt to taste and stir to combine well.

2.Divide the pork mixture between dumplings. Moisten the edge of each dumpling with water, fold the top half over the bottom half and press together firmly.

3.Place your dumplings in the Air Fryer cooking basket and spritz them with cooking spray. Cook your dumplings at 400 degrees F for 8 minutes. Work with batches.

4.While your dumplings are cooking, whisk the sauce ingredients. Serve the warm dumplings with the sauce for dipping. Enjoy!

Mexican-Style Corn on the Cob with Bacon

Cooking Time:

20 minutes

Serve: 3

Ingredients:

2 slices bacon
4 ears fresh corn, shucked and cut into halves
1 avocado, pitted, peeled and mashed
1 teaspoon ancho chili powder
2 garlic cloves
2 tablespoons cilantro, chopped
1 teaspoon lime juice
Salt and black pepper, to taste

Directions:

1. Start by preheating your Air Fryer to 400 degrees F. Cook the bacon for 6 to 7 minutes; chop into small chunks and reserve. Spritz the corn with cooking spray.

2. Cook at 395 degrees F for 8 minutes, turning them over halfway through the cooking time. Mix the reserved bacon with the remaining ingredients.

3. Spoon the bacon mixture over the corn on the cob and serve immediately.

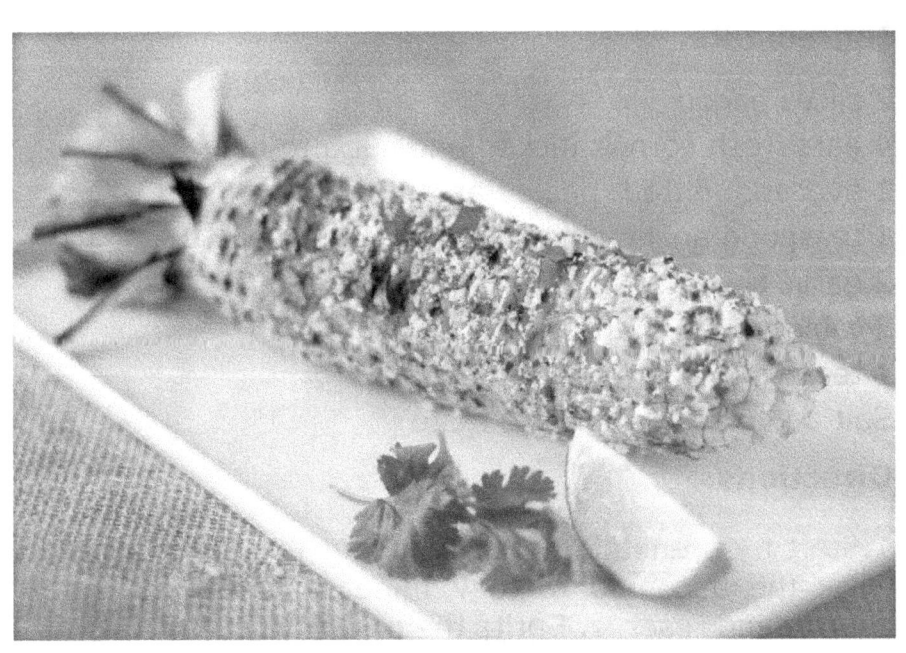

Mini Plantain Cups

Cooking Time:

10 minutes

Serve: 3

Ingredients:

2 blackened plantains, chopped
¼ cup all-purpose flour
½ cup cornmeal
½ cup milk
1 tablespoon coconut oil
1 teaspoon fresh ginger, peeled and minced
A pinch of salt
A pinch of ground cinnamon

Directions:

1. In a mixing bowl, thoroughly combine all ingredients until everything is well incorporated. Spoon the batter into a greased mini muffin tin.

2. Bake the mini plantain cups in your Air Fryer at 330 degrees F for 6 to 7 minutes or until golden brown. Enjoy!

Sweet Potato Fries with Spicy Dip

Cooking Time:

50 minutes

Serve: 3

Ingredients:

2 medium sweet potatoes, cut into

⅓ -inch sticks

2 tablespoons olive oil

1 teaspoon kosher salt

Spicy Dip: ¼ cup mayonnaise

¼ cup Greek yogurt

¼ teaspoon Dijon mustard

1 teaspoon hot sauce

Directions:

1. Soak the sweet potato in icy cold water for 30 minutes. Drain the sweet potatoes and pat them dry with paper towels.

2. Toss the sweet potatoes with olive oil and salt. Place in the lightly greased cooking basket.

3. Cook in the preheated Air Fryer at 360 degrees F for 14 minutes. Wok in batches.

4.While the sweet potatoes are cooking, make the spicy dip by whisking the remaining ingredients. Place in the refrigerator until ready to serve. Enjoy!

The Best Calamari Appetizer

Cooking Time:

20 minutes

Serve: 6

Ingredients

1½ pounds calamari tubes, cleaned, cut into rings
Sea salt and ground black pepper, to taste
2 tablespoons lemon juice
1 cup cornmeal
1 cup all-purpose flour
1 teaspoon paprika
1 egg, whisked
¼ cup buttermilk

Directions:

1. Preheat your Air Fryer to 390 degrees F. Rinse the calamari and pat it dry. Season with salt and black pepper.

2. Drizzle lemon juice all over the calamari. Now, combine the cornmeal, flour, and paprika in a bowl; add the whisked egg and buttermilk. Dredge the calamari in the egg/flour mixture.

3. Arrange them in the cooking basket. Spritz with cooking oil and cook for 9 to 12 minutes, shaking the basket occasionally. Work in batches. Serve with toothpicks. Enjoy!

The Best Party Mix Ever

Cooking Time:

25 minutes

Serve: 4

Ingredients:

1cups mini pretzels
1 cup mini crackers
1 cup peanuts
1 tablespoon Creole seasoning
2 tablespoons butter, melted

Directions:

1.Toss all ingredients in the Air Fryer basket. Cook in the preheated Air Fryer at 360 degrees F approximately 9 minutes until lightly toasted.

2.Shake the basket periodically. Enjoy!

Cocktail Sausage and Veggies on a Stick

Cooking Time:

25 minutes

Serve: 6

Ingredients:

16 cocktail sausages, halved
16 pearl onions
1 red bell pepper, cut into 1 ½-inch pieces
1 green bell pepper, cut into 1 ½-inch pieces
Salt and cracked black pepper, to taste
½ cup tomato chili sauce

Directions

1. Thread the cocktail sausages, pearl onions, and peppers alternately onto skewers. Sprinkle with salt and black pepper.

2. Cook in the preheated Air Fryer at 380 degrees for 15 minutes, turning the skewers over once or twice to ensure even cooking. Serve with the tomato chili sauce on the side. Enjoy!

Red Beet Chips with Pizza Sauce

Cooking Time:

30 minutes

Serve: 4

Ingredients:

1 red beets, thinly sliced
1 tablespoon grapeseed oil
1 teaspoon seasoned salt
½ teaspoon ground black pepper
¼ teaspoon cumin powder
½ cup pizza sauce

Directions:

1. Toss the red beets with the oil, salt, black pepper, and cumin powder.

2. Arrange the beet slices in a single layer in the Air Fryer basket.

3. Cook in the preheated Air Fryer at 330 degrees F for 13 minutes. Serve with the pizza sauce and enjoy!

Fried Pickle Chips with Greek Yogurt Dip

Cooking Time:

20 minutes

Serve: 5

Ingredients:

½ cup cornmeal
½ cup all-purpose flour
1 teaspoon cayenne pepper
½ teaspoon shallot powder
1 teaspoon garlic powder
½ teaspoon porcini powder
Kosher salt and ground black pepper, to taste
2 eggs
2 cups pickle chips, pat dry with kitchen towels

Greek Yogurt Dip:

½ cup Greek yogurt

1 clove garlic, minced

¼ teaspoon ground black pepper

1 tablespoon fresh chives, chopped

Directions:

1.In a shallow bowl, mix the cornmeal and flour; add the seasonings and mix to combine well. Beat the eggs in a separate shallow bowl.

2.Dredge the pickle chips in the flour mixture, then, in the egg mixture.

3. Press the pickle chips into the flour mixture again, coating evenly. Cook in the preheated Air Fryer at 400 degrees F for 5 minutes; shake the basket and cook for 5 minutes more.

4.Work in batches. Meanwhile, mix all the sauce ingredients until well combined. Serve the fried pickles with the Greek yogurt dip and enjoy.

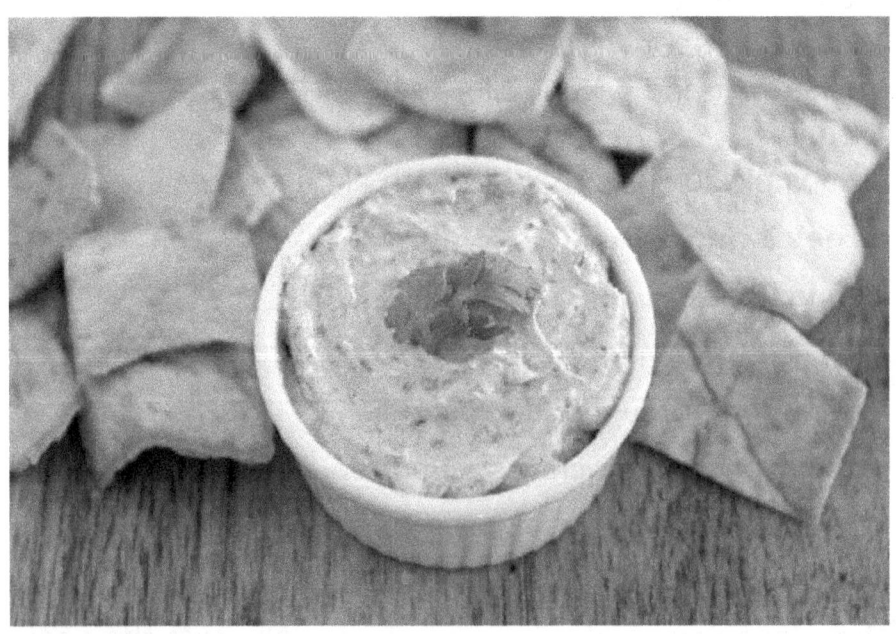

Parmesan Squash Chips

Cooking Time:

20 minutes

Serve: 3

Ingredients:

¾ pound butternut squash, cut into thin rounds
½ cup Parmesan cheese, grated
Sea salt and ground black pepper, to taste
1 teaspoon butter
½ cup ketchup
1 teaspoon Sriracha sauce

Directions:

1. Toss the butternut squash with Parmesan cheese, salt, black pepper and butter. Transfer the butternut squash rounds to the Air Fryer cooking basket.

2. Air Fryer at 400 degrees F for 12 minutes. Shake the Air Fryer basket periodically to ensure even cooking. Work with batches.

3. While the parmesan squash chips are baking, whisk the ketchup and sriracha and set it aside. Serve the parmesan squash chips with Sriracha ketchup and enjoy!

Hot Paprika Bacon Deviled Eggs

Cooking Time:

15 minutes

Serve: 4

Ingredients:

4 eggs
2 ounces bacon bits
2 tablespoons mayonnaise
2 tablespoons cream cheese
1 teaspoon hot sauce
½ teaspoon garlic, minced
1 tablespoon pickle relish
½ teaspoon hot paprika
Salt and ground black pepper, to taste

Directions:

1. Place the wire rack in the Air Fryer basket and lower the eggs onto the rack.

2. Cook the eggs at 260 degrees F for 15 minutes. Transfer the eggs to an ice-cold water bath to stop cooking.

3. Peel the eggs under cold running water; slice them into halves, separating the whites and yolks.

4. Mash the egg yolks; add in the remaining ingredients

and stir to combine; spoon the yolk mixture into the egg whites. Serve and enjoy!

Kid-Friendly Mozzarella Sticks

Cooking Time:

10 minutes

Serve: 3

Ingredients:

2 eggs
¼ cup corn flour
¼ cup plain flour
1 cup Italian-style dried breadcrumbs
1 teaspoon Italian seasoning mix
10 ounces mozzarella, cut into
½-inch sticks
1 cup marinara sauce

Directions:

1. Beat the eggs in a shallow bowl until pale and frothy. Then, in a second bowl, place both types of flour.

2. In a third bowl, mix breadcrumbs with Italian seasoning mix. Dip the mozzarella sticks in the beaten eggs and allow the excess egg to drip back into the bowl.

3. Then, dip the mozzarella sticks in the flour mixture. Lastly, roll them over the seasoned breadcrumbs. Cook the mozzarella sticks in the preheated Air Fryer at 370 degrees F for 4 minutes.

4.Flip them over and continue to cook for 2 to 3 minutes more. Serve the mozzarella sticks with marinara sauce. Enjoy!

www.ingramcontent.com/pod-product-compliance
Lightning Source LLC
Chambersburg PA
CBHW071112030426
42336CB00013BA/2047